Mommy has a Boo-Boo Now What?

A Guided Journal For Parents & Children
To Help Cope With Breast Cancer

Mommy has a Boo-Boo Now What?

ISBN: 978-1-7367038-1-6

Hi Parents!

As I went through my own journey my children had a lot of questions. I hope this guided journal/coloring book will bring awareness and help your child cope while you are getting treated. There are questions in here they might be afraid to ask and with your assistance you can help them.

With Love,

MARCI GREENBERG COX

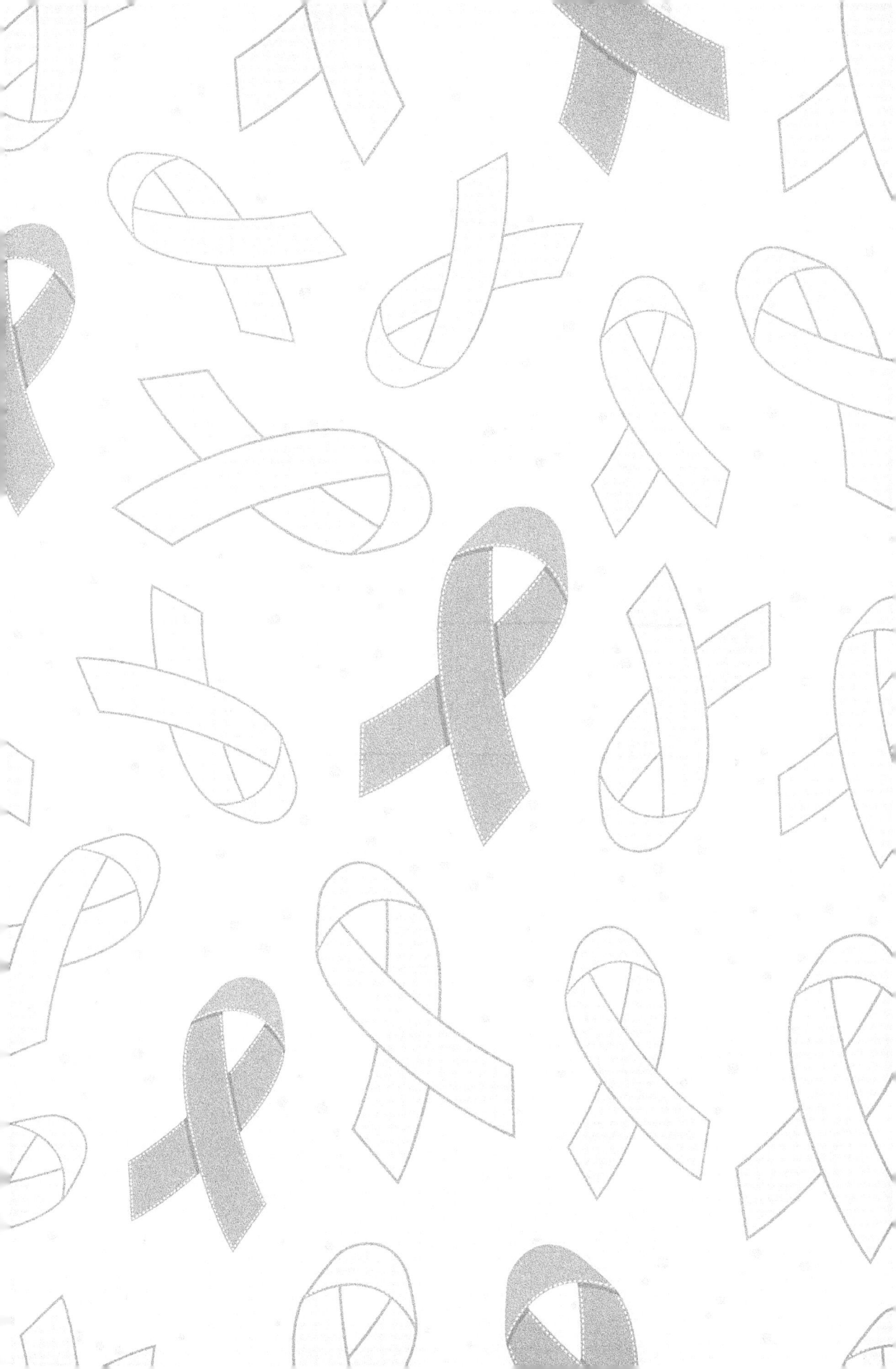

This book belongs to:

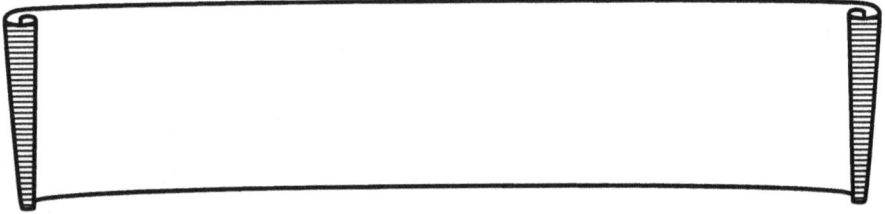

Where is the boo-boo?

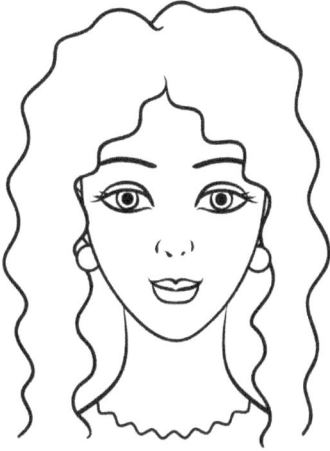

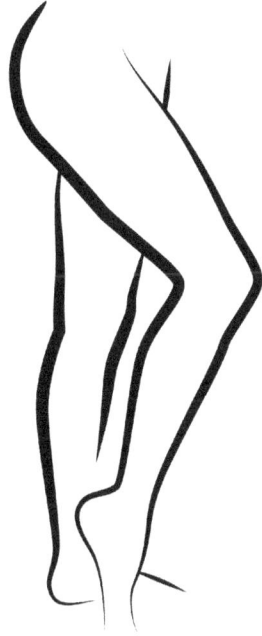

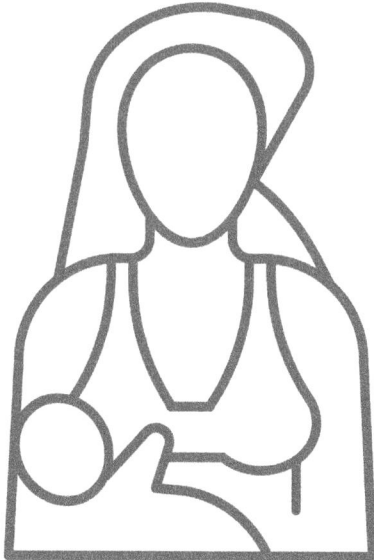

Does the boo-boo
make you scared?

Why or why not?

Is there a name for it?
What is it called?

circle one

yes   no

Can you catch cancer like you catch a cold?

circle one

yes   no

Can I get cancer from you?

circle one

yes   no

Why did you get a boo-boo?

have a discussion

Who will take care of me while you are getting better?

_____

_____

_____

Who is going to take me to school?

_____

_____

_____

Who is going to take me to: sports, dance, music lesson, etc?

_____

_____

_____

Is it okay if
I do not want to play
with my friends?
Is that normal?

circle one

yes   no

yes   no

Mommy is seeing the doctor today how do you feel?

color one

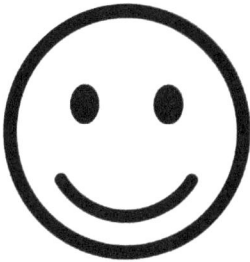 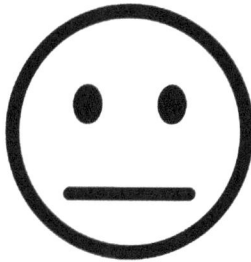 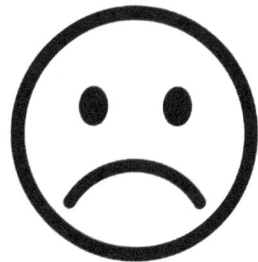

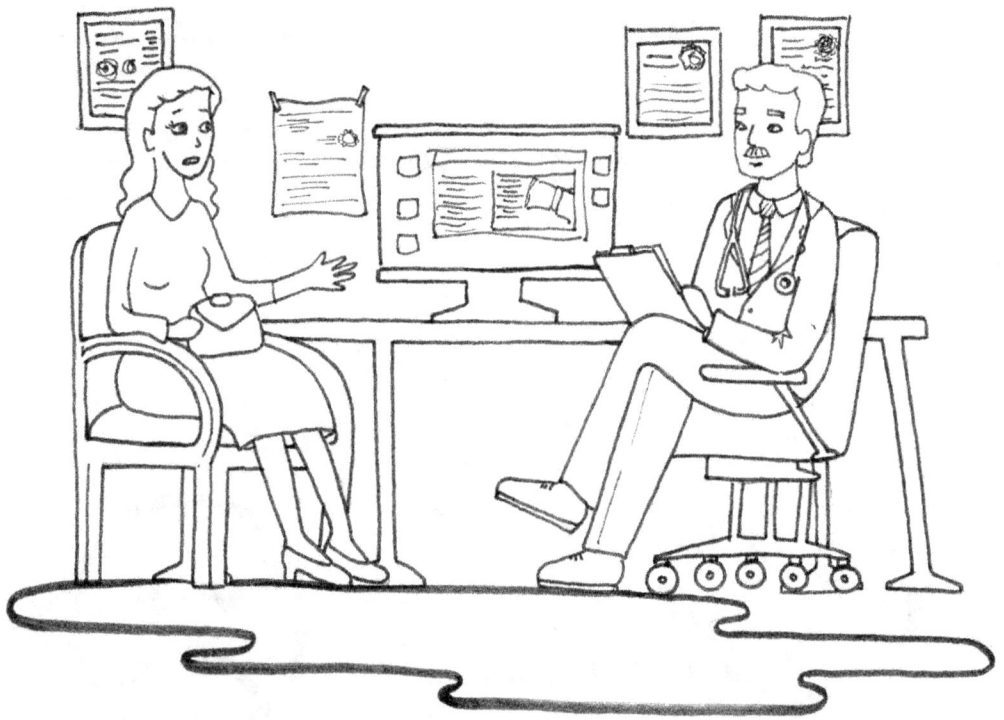

Mommy has to take
medicine and go every few
weeks. She might be very
tired and get sick. How
can you help Mommy?

draw or write

Keep drawing or writing

Some mommies have to
have chemotherapy.
What is chemotherapy?

have a discussion

If Mommy has to have chemo -
how long is chemo?

_____

_____

_____

If Mommy has to have chemo -
how often do you have to go?

_____

_____

_____

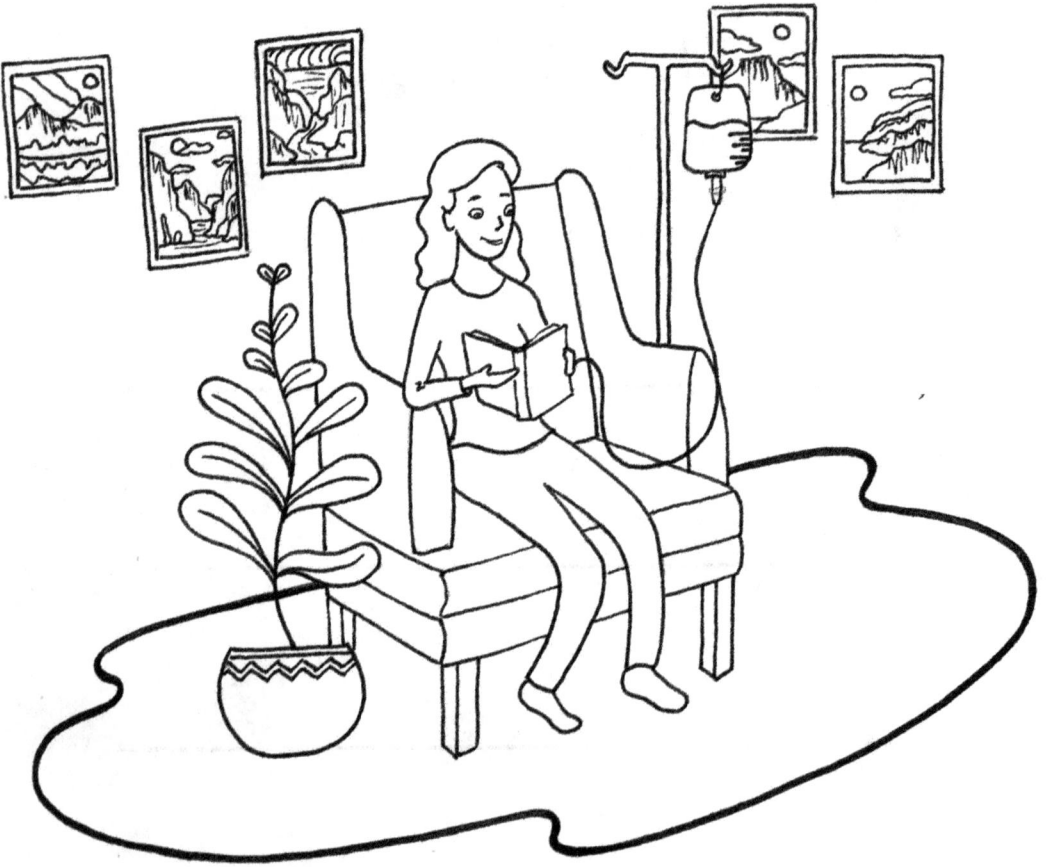

Mommy is having surgery today.
How do you feel?

color one

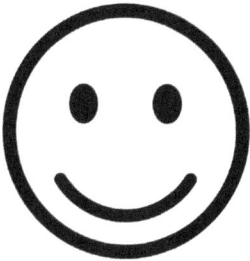 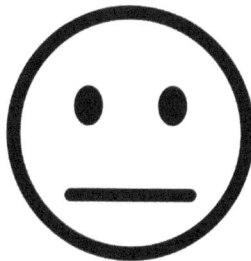 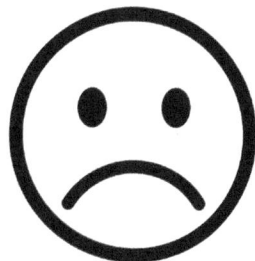

What type of surgery is Mommy having?

circle one

lumpectomy or mastectomy?

have a discussion
on what you are having
and what it means.

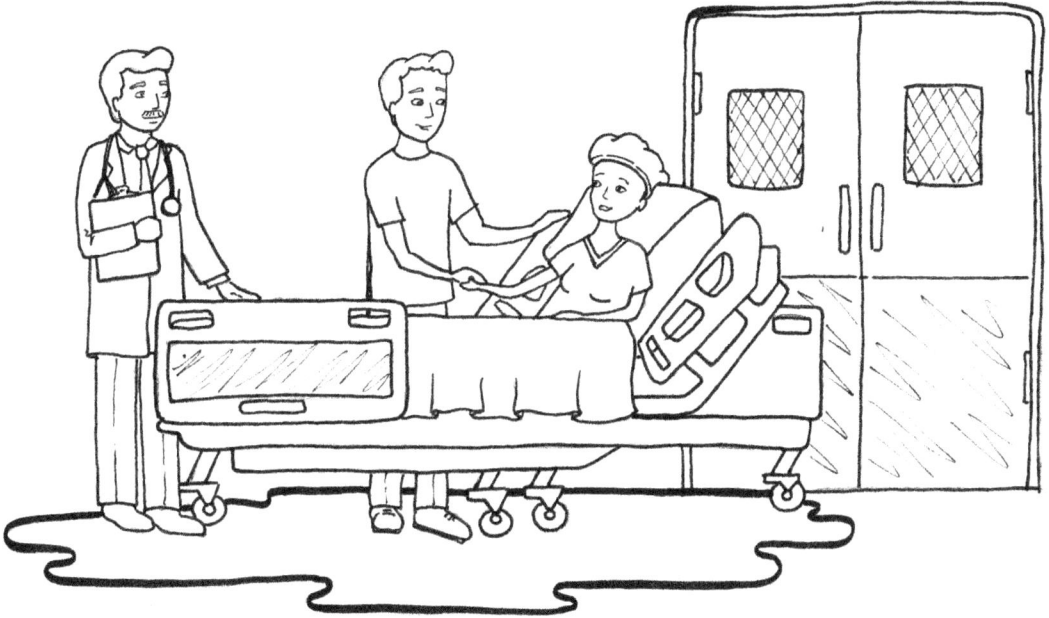
OPERATING ROOM

If Mommy's boobies are gone, how do you feel?

color one

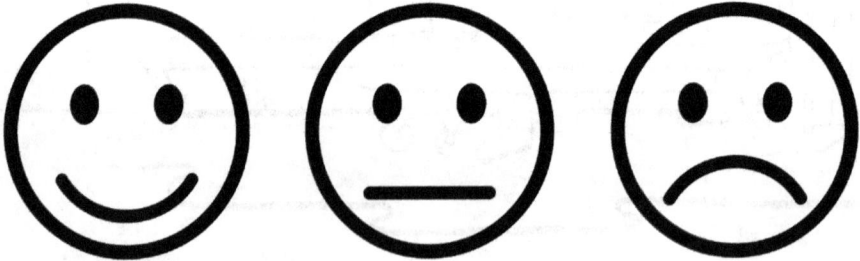

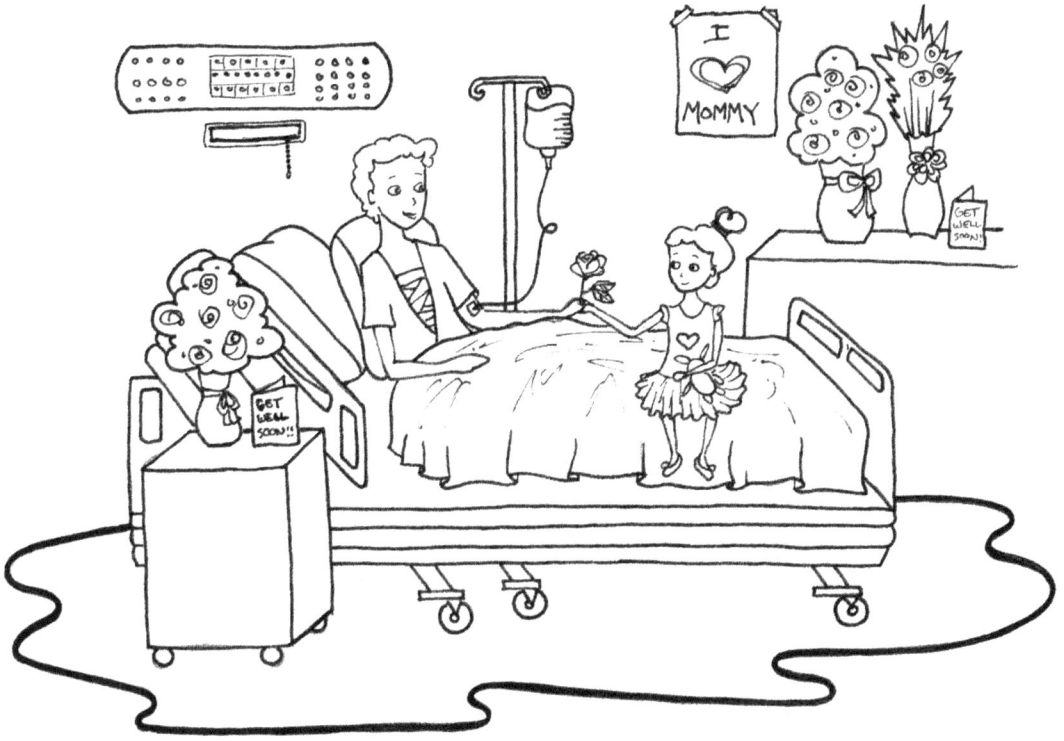

Should Mommy get new boobies?

circle one

yes   no

If Mommy decides not
to get new boobies that
means she will
stay flat.
How do you feel?

color one

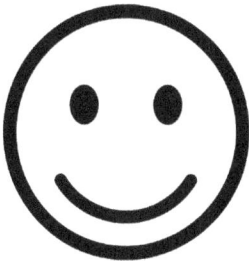 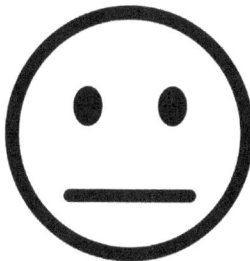 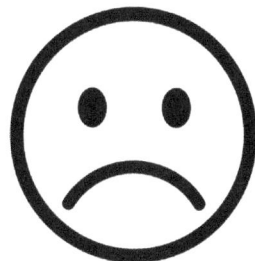

Are you afraid to look at Mommy's scars?

circle one

yes   no

Mommy is home and healing. She is hurting and can't hold you. How can you help her?

draw or write

Keep drawing or writing

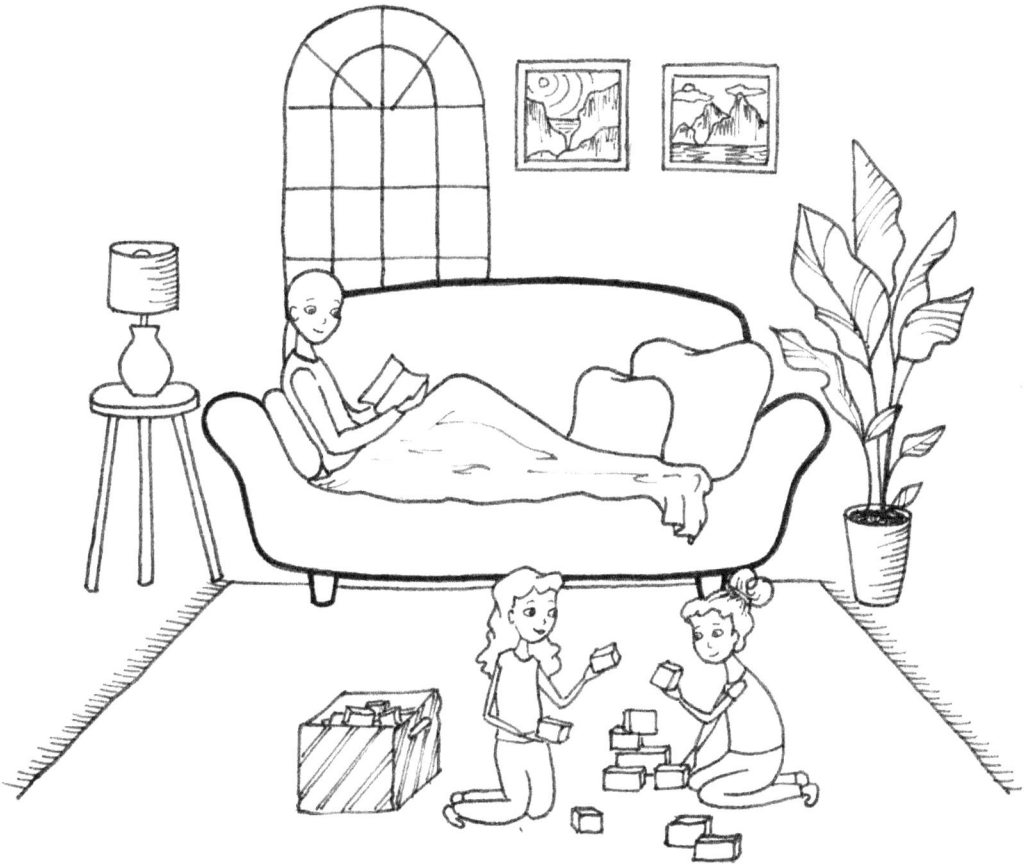

Mommy is starting to
lose her hair.
How does that
make you feel?

color one

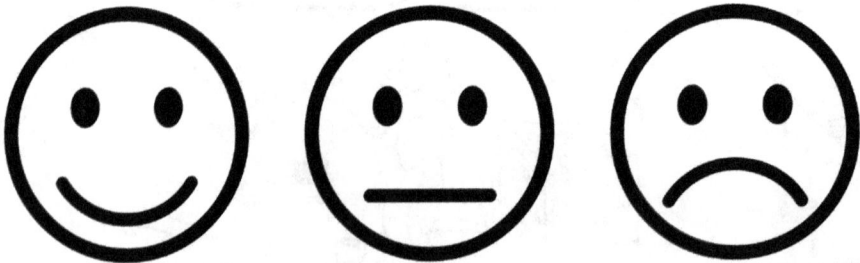

Why did you lose your hair?

have a discussion

Will your hair grow back?

circle one

yes   no

What can you do to help Mommy feel better about losing her hair?

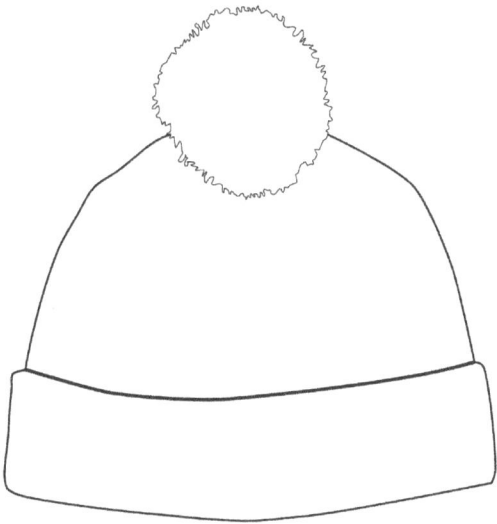

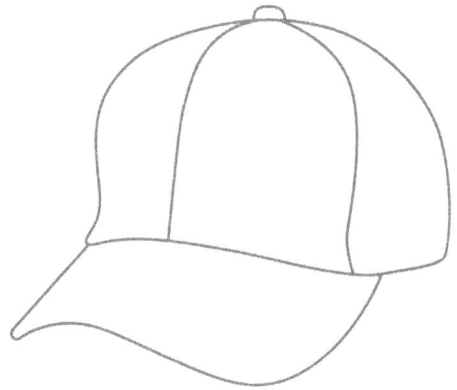

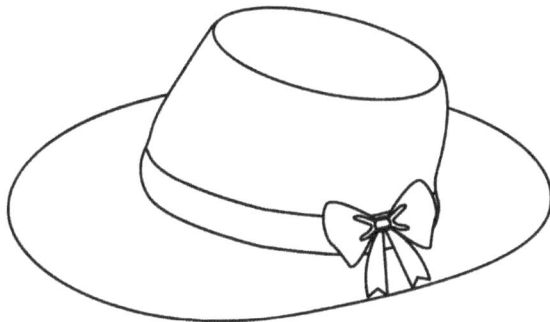

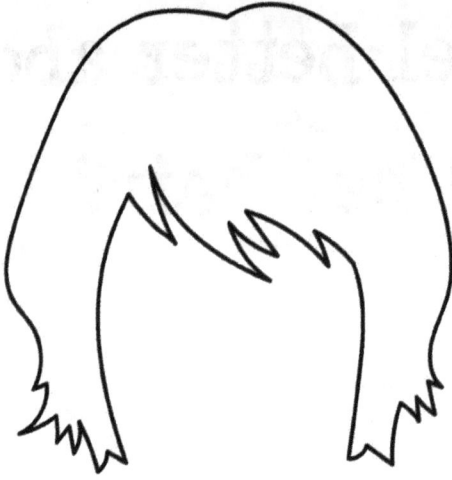

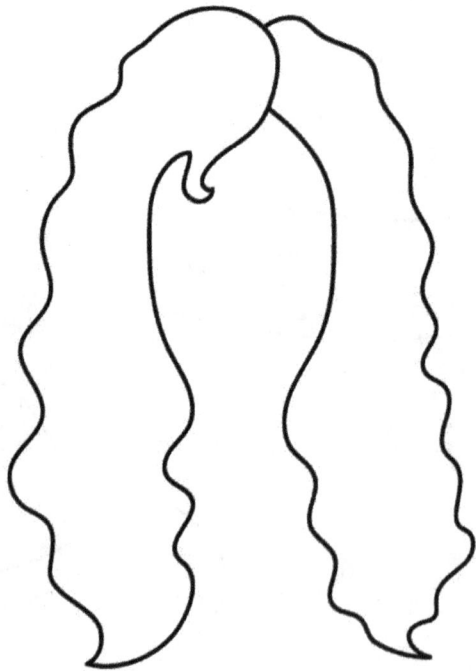

Draw your own ideas
to help Mommy

Mommy might have to have radiation.
What is radiation?

have a discussion

If Mommy has to have radiation -
how long is radiation?

_____

_____

_____

If Mommy has to have
radiation -
how often do
you have to
have radiation?

_____

_____

_____

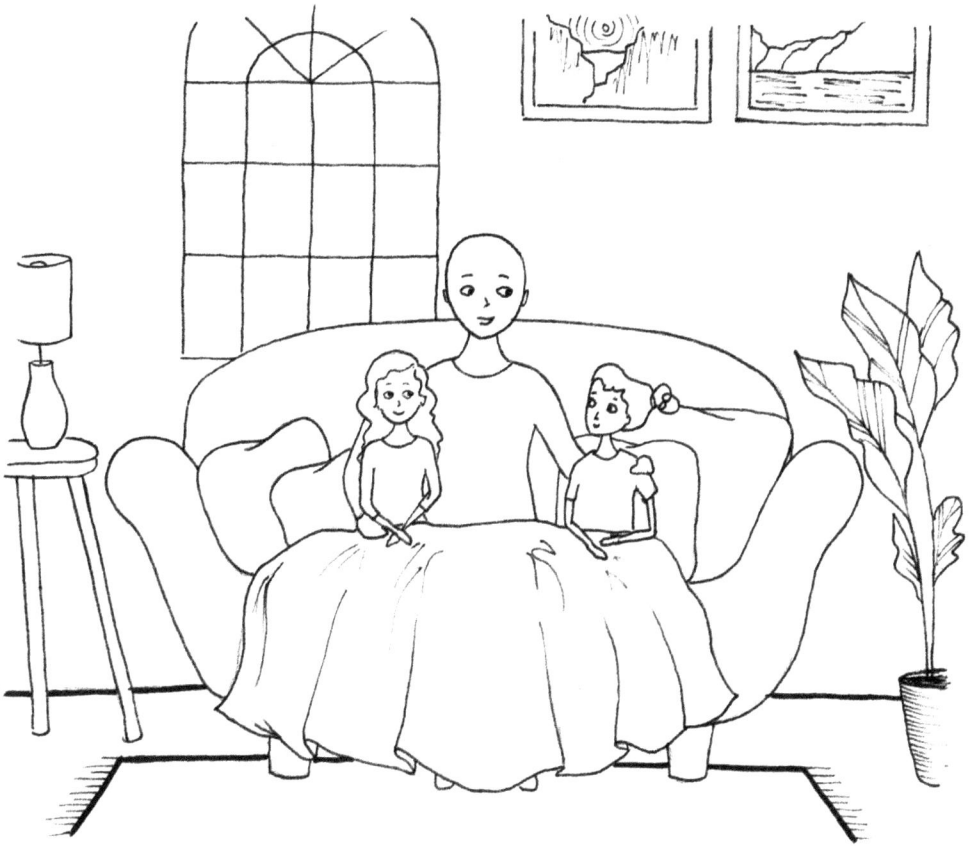

What makes you happy?

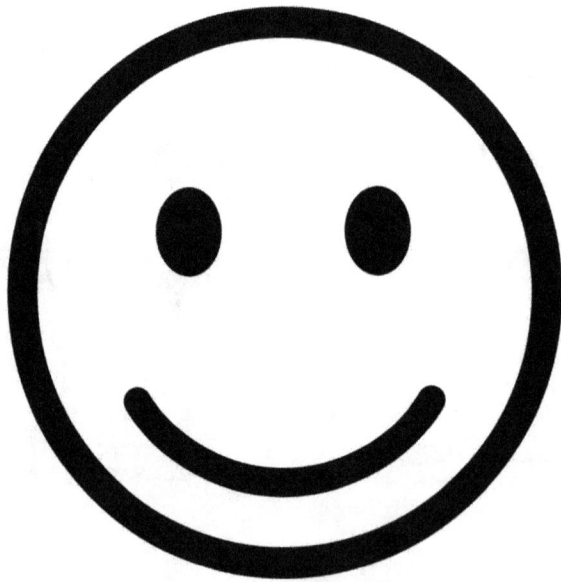

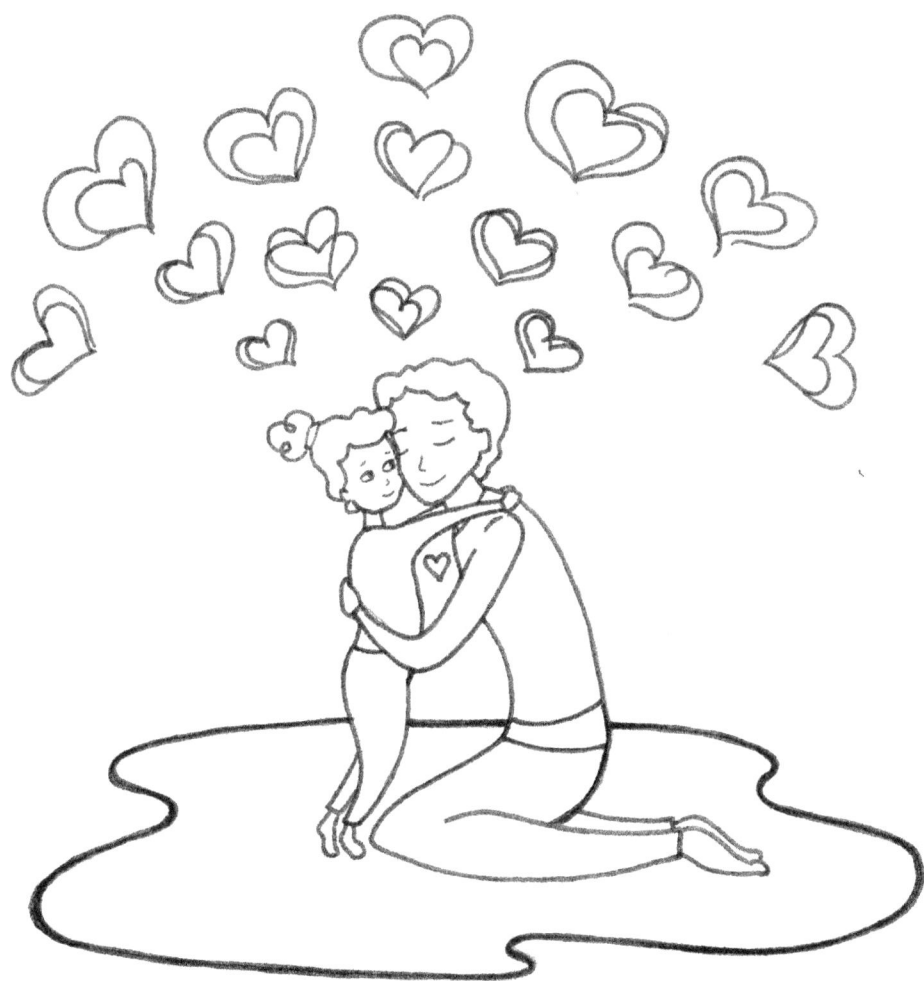

What makes you sad?

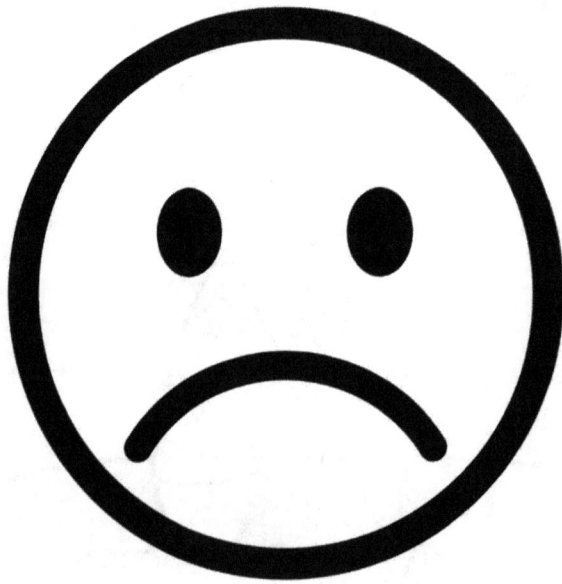

Draw or write what makes you sad

Can the cancer
come back?

circle one

yes   no

If I want to talk
to someone
who can I talk to?

_____

_____

_____

Are you going to die?

have a discussion

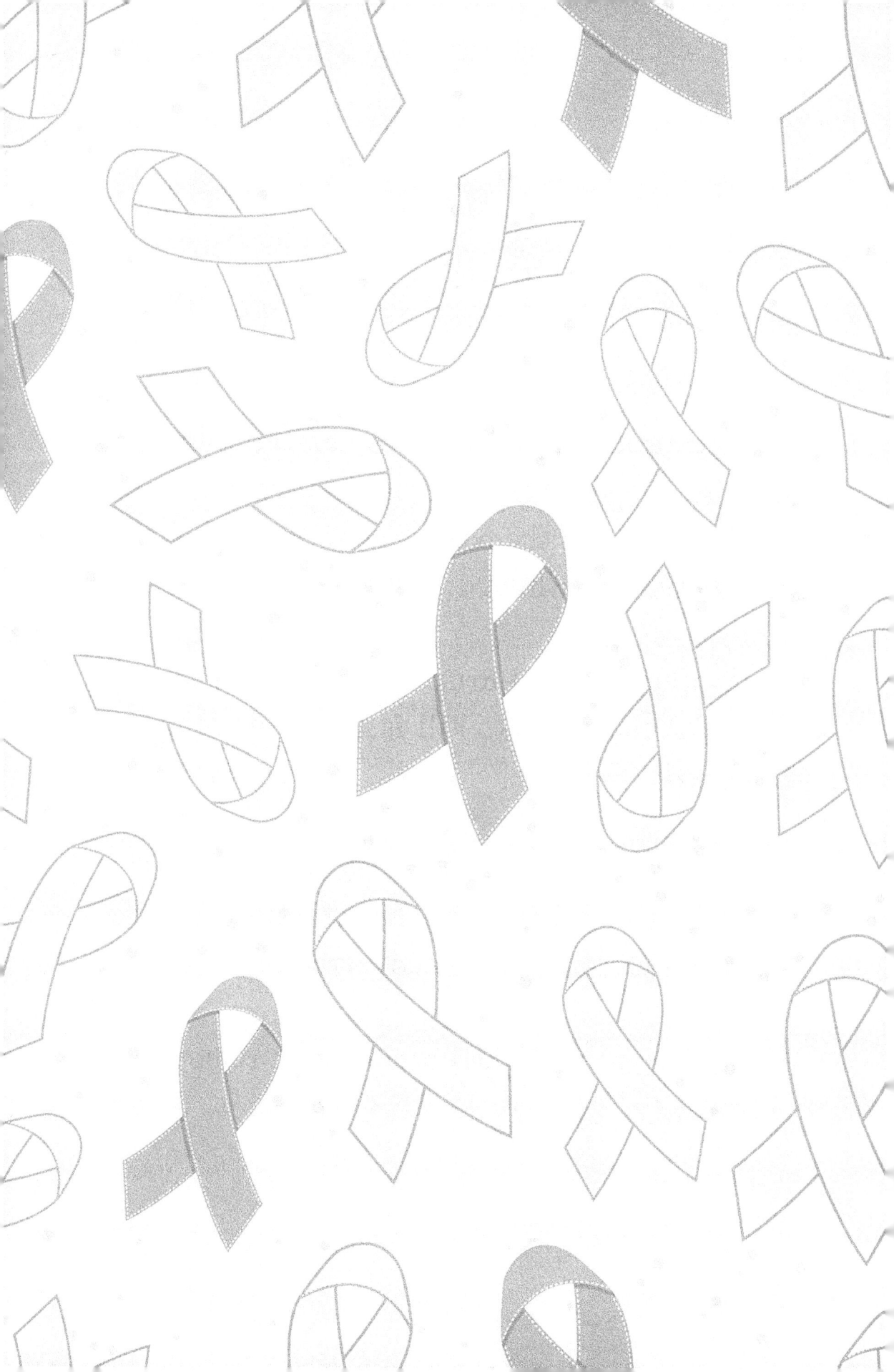

List of Cancer Words and the meanings:

<u>Cancer</u> - is a group of diseases involving abnormal cell growth with the potential to invade or spread to other parts of the body. These contrast with benign tumors, which do not spread

<u>Chemotherapy</u> - is a drug treatment that uses powerful chemicals to kill fast-growing cells in your body.

<u>Lumpectomy</u> - a surgical operation in which a lump is removed from the breast, typically when cancer is present but has not spread.

<u>Mastectomy</u> - a surgical operation to remove a breast.

Radiation therapy - (also called radiotherapy) is a cancer treatment that uses high doses of radiation to kill cancer cells and shrink tumors.

Surgery - the branch of medical practice that treats injuries, diseases, and deformities by the physical removal, repair, or readjustment of organs and tissues, often involving cutting into the body.

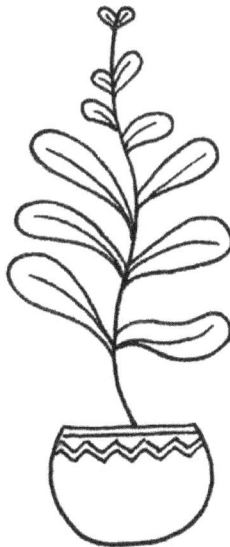